Contents

INTRODUCTION	5
CHAPTER ONE	7
What is Soluble Fiber?	9
Health Benefits of Soluble Fiber	9
Foods High in Soluble Fiber	10
What is Insoluble Fiber?	11
Soluble Fiber Vs. Insoluble Fiber	11
Health Benefits of Insoluble Fiber	12
Foods High in Insoluble Fiber	12
What is Prebiotic Fiber?	13
Health Benefits of Prebiotic Fiber	14
What are the Best High Fiber Foods?	15
What is a High Fiber Diet?	18
High Fiber Fruits	19
High Fiber Vegetables	20
High Fiber Grains	21
High Fiber Supplements	22
What other things does fiber do?	24
Dangers and Side Effects	25
How much fiber should I eat?	26
Tips for increasing dietary fiber in your diet:	28

CHAPTER TWO 30

High-Fiber Diet Meal Plan 30

Diet Plan If You Want Weight Loss 31

Diet Plan for Adding Muscle Mass 32

A Typical High-Fiber Week 34

Recipe for All Plans 36

Spicy Skillet Chicken 37

Slow-Cooker Black Beans and Rice 39

Lemon Cake Pops 41

Pasta and Bean Skillet 42

Mocha Coffee Frappé 43

Steamed Chinese Vegetables with Brown Rice 44

Grilled Barbecued Beef and Bean Burgers 46

Red Bean and Rice Cakes 48

Lentil-Vegetable Soup 51

Chocolate Fudge Brownie Berry Sundae 53

Mexican Chocolate Cream Pie 53

Lemon Strawberry Shortcake Trifle 55

Chicken and Northern Beans White Chili 56

Vegetarian Vegetable and Bean Chili 58

Oatmeal Raisin Cookie Ice Cream Sandwich 61

Dutch Oven Black Bean Soup 62

Mini Peanut Butter Brownie Cupcake 64

Frozen Yogurt Cookie Sundae 66
Upside Down Lemon Cream Pie 67
Mango Lemon Leche 68
Chocolate and Pear Coffee Cake 69
Cinnamon and Lime Chicken Fajitas 70
Fiery Fish Tacos with Crunchy Corn Salsa 72
Quinoa and Black Beans 75
Simple Baked Beans 77
Wendy's Quick Pasta and Lentils 78
Whole Wheat Pasta 80
Chinese Chicken Salad III 81
Irish Chicken and Dumplings 84
Vegetarian Chickpea Sandwich Filling 86
Greek Chicken Pasta 87
Red Lentil Curry 90
Chickpea Curry 92
Southwest Chicken 94
Slow Cooker Chicken Cacciatore 95
Black Beans and Rice 97
Easy Red Beans and Rice 98
Slow Cooker Chicken Marrakesh 100
Garlic Chicken Stir Fry 102
Greek Pasta with Tomatoes and White Beans 104

CONCLUSION 106

INTRODUCTION

Many people enjoy the health benefits of a high-fiber diet. A specialized diet can help address many physical ailments, and eating foods with high fiber content reduces blood-cholesterol levels while aiding in the normalization of sugar levels in the bloodstream. This promotes greater overall health and can be a valuable asset in any weight-loss program. By normalizing your blood-sugar levels, you avoid the crash often felt when eating sugary or greasy foods. This can give you the energy you need to tackle the next workout on your schedule and feel great throughout the day. While the plan may offer some difficulty when it comes to meal planning, it is fairly simple to follow.

Healthy fiber-rich foods help you feel full, support your digestive system, and make achieving your weight loss goals a lot easier.

Thanks to the highly-refined, modern American diet, the average American isn't getting enough of one of the most important nutrients: fiber. Without a consistent intake of healthy, soluble and insoluble high-fiber foods in your diet, you'll experience dips in energy, have difficulty losing weight, and also increase your risk of diabetes and inflammation.

CHAPTER ONE

Fiber is a complex carbohydrate found in the cell walls of all plant-based foods. While the body converts other carbohydrates such as starch into simple sugars for energy, it's not able to fully break down fiber. Fiber actually passes through most of your body's digestive system undigested until it reaches the large intestine, or colon. Depending on its function in the digestive system, fiber can be soluble, insoluble, or prebiotic, and is found in these categories of plant-based foods:

- Fruit

- Vegetables

- Whole grains

- Legumes

- Nuts and Seeds

A high fiber diet packs many impressive health benefits. Eating more fiber can help you maintain a healthy weight by keeping you full and reducing the chance of overeating. Adding more fiber to your diet can help lower cholesterol, which may prevent chronic diseases such as type 2 diabetes and heart disease. High fiber foods may also reduce the risk of certain cancers and promote a healthy gut by helping waste to pass through your digestive system efficiently. Our high fiber diet guide teaches you everything you need to know about this heart-healthy way of eating, including how to identify the best sources of fiber. Our sample high fiber meal plan includes recipes for breakfasts, snacks, and more, so you can jump start a fresh routine to better health.

What is Soluble Fiber?

When soluble fiber enters our digestive system, it dissolves in water and takes on a viscous, gelatinous form. This type of fiber is typically derived from the inner flesh of plant-based foods. In the large intestine, soluble fibers such as pectin (the same "pectin" found in jams and jellies), inulin, gum, mucilage, and beta glucan mix with partially digested foods to help them pass more efficiently.

Health Benefits of Soluble Fiber

Soluble fiber promotes a healthy heart by regulating cholesterol levels in the body and by lowering blood pressure. For example, pectin helps limit the amount of fat your body absorbs from certain foods, while beta glucan is strongly linked to lowering bad cholesterol. Soluble fiber can also be very beneficial to those with type 2 diabetes by helping to lower and regulate blood glucose levels. A healthier blood glucose level may also lead to a reduced need for insulin in some diabetics.

Foods High in Soluble Fiber

Soluble fiber is often associated with the flesh or pulp of foods such as potatoes and oranges. Depending on the food, cooking can make the consistency soft and mushy—think oatmeal, baked pears, or boiled sweet potatoes.

- Whole-grain oats

- Barley

- Black beans

- Lentils

- Raspberries

- Apples

- Sweet potatoes

- Oranges

What is Insoluble Fiber?

Insoluble fiber retains water once it enters the digestive system and sweeps waste through the large intestine. This type of fiber is derived from a plant's tough, outer skin and is made up of cellulose and lignin molecules. Typically, you'll find insoluble fiber in the skins of fruits and vegetables such as apples, pears, and potatoes.

Soluble Fiber Vs. Insoluble Fiber

From apples to potatoes, every type of plant has a protective cell wall that provides shape and texture. Inside a plant's cell wall are fiber molecules that strengthen and support growth. When the plant is eaten, these fibers enter our digestive system and become either soluble or insoluble. The main distinction between these two types of fibers is their ability to dissolve in water. While soluble fiber combines with food in the large intestine, insoluble fiber acts more like a digestive "broom."

Health Benefits of Insoluble Fiber

Insoluble fiber prevents constipation and complications such as hemorrhoids by bulking up the stool, helping it pass more quickly through the intestines. Insoluble fiber may also help decrease the risk for colorectal cancer by speeding up waste's movement through the digestive tract. The shorter the amount of time waste spends in your body, the less of chance there is for harmful substances to pass through your intestinal walls into the bloodstream.

Foods High in Insoluble Fiber

Foods packed with insoluble fiber often have a tough or chewy texture—think fruit and vegetable skins, and wheat bran, the hard outer layer of cereal grains. Here are several top sources of insoluble fiber:

• Whole-wheat bread

• Wheat bran

- Corn

- Brussels sprouts

- Apples

- Kidney beans

What is Prebiotic Fiber?

Some soluble fibers such as pectin, beta glucan, and inulin are prebiotic, meaning they can be fermented into energy sources for the good bacteria, or probiotics, in your large intestine. Your large intestine houses more bacteria—both good and bad—than any other part of your body. Prebiotics keep bad bacteria at bay by feeding probiotics, which contributes to a healthier microbiome and better overall health.

Health Benefits of Prebiotic Fiber

Think of your relationship with your gut as symbiotic. Eat more prebiotic fiber to help the good bacteria thrive, and they will give back by providing key health benefits. Specifically, prebiotics such as inulin produce short-chain fatty acids that help the body better absorb essential minerals—calcium, iron, and magnesium. These fatty acids may also protect against inflammation, lower cholesterol, and reduce the risk for colorectal cancer. Prebiotics may also help boost overall immunity.

Foods High in Prebiotic Fiber:

• Chicory root

• Dandelion root

• Globe artichoke

• Onions and leeks

- Garlic

- Barley

- Bananas

What are the Best High Fiber Foods?

Below, find some of the best high fiber fruits, vegetables, legumes, grains, nuts, and seeds to meet your daily requirements more easily. While there is technically no set maximum amount of fiber that you can consume at each meal or during the day, keep in mind that too much may cause bloating and stomach pain.

Serving Size Calories Fiber (grams)

Legumes

Split peas, cooked 1/2 cup 116 8.1

Lentils, cooked 1/2 cup 115 5.5

Black beans, cooked 1/2 cup 114 7.5

Chickpeas, cooked 1/2 cup 135 6.2

Vegetables

Artichoke hearts, cooked 1 each 60 6.5

Sweet potato, baked, with skin 1 medium 105 3.8

Pumpkin, canned 1/2 cup 42 3.6

Broccoli, cooked 1/2 cup 27 2.6

Fruits

Apple, with skin 1 small 77 3.6

Raspberries 1/2 cup 32 4.0

Banana 1 medium 105 3.1

Figs, dried 1/4 cup 93 3.7

Grains

Quinoa, cooked 1/2 cup 111 2.6

Bulgur, cooked 1/2 cup 76 4.1

Pearled barley, cooked 1/2 cup 97 3.0

Oatmeal, cooked 1/2 cup 83 2.0

Nuts/Seeds

Almonds 1 ounce 164 3.5

Chia seeds, dry 1 tablespoon 69 4.9

Pistachios 1 ounce 160 3.0

Walnuts 1 ounce 185 1.9

What is a High Fiber Diet?

Because fiber is only found in plant-based foods, you should naturally find yourself eating less meat on a high fiber diet. Additionally, many of the best fiber sources are whole (or minimally-processed), nutrient-dense foods. A high fiber diet also promotes healthier eating patterns overall. High fiber foods such as whole grains, fruits, vegetables, nuts, and seeds can take longer to chew than other foods and will help keep you full longer. Add more fiber-rich foods into your diet to help you eat slower, savor your meals, and prevent overeating.

If you're just starting a high fiber diet, it's important to increase your fiber intake gradually, as too much too quickly can cause an upset stomach. Drinking plenty of fluids can help keep waste moving through your digestive tract smoothly, too. It should take only a couple of weeks for your body to adjust to a higher intake of fiber, and once it does you'll be able to experience its many benefits.

To get the most benefits from a high fiber diet, you should be consuming a variety of fiber-rich fruits, vegetables, legumes, grains, nuts, and seeds over the course of the day. Just because bananas are a good source of fiber doesn't mean you should be eating 10 of them to meet your daily needs. Doing so will cause you to miss out on other key nutrients that come from a diverse high fiber diet. Here's a breakdown of the high fiber diet's top players, and why it's important to incorporate foods from each category into your daily routine.

High Fiber Fruits

Skin-on fruits, such as apples and pears, tend to have higher amounts of insoluble fiber, while softer varieties, such as raspberries and bananas, are higher in soluble fiber. Fruit juice is not a good source of fiber, as it's usually made without the peel or pulp. One cup of orange juice contains 0.5 grams of fiber, while 1 medium orange packs about 3 grams. Fruit is also a valuable source for antioxidants, potassium, folate, and key vitamins and minerals. Here are several (of many) high fiber fruits:

- Apples

- Oranges

- Bananas

- Raspberries, blueberries, strawberries

- Mangos

High Fiber Vegetables

Like fruits, vegetables are also a low-calorie fiber source and should be consumed with the skin on when possible. Comparatively, ½ cup of mashed potatoes has 1.6 grams of fiber, while a small baked potato has 3.2 grams (over twice as much!). Vegetables also contain many of the same health perks as fruits, packing antioxidants, vitamins, and minerals. See below for a list of high fiber vegetables:

- Artichokes

- Brussels sprouts

- Broccoli

- Collard greens, kale, beet greens, Swiss chard

- Carrots, parsnips, turnips, celery root, beets

High Fiber Grains
Always choose whole grains over refined to make sure you're getting the most fiber. Incorporating more whole grain foods, which are often calorie-dense, onto your plate can help prevent overeating. Wheat bran contains about 12 grams per ½ cup serving, and is often added to cereals,

breads, and baked goods to boost fiber. You can also purchase wheat bran (also called millers bran) whole and sprinkle it over yogurt and salads. Additionally, whole grains can provide selenium, iron, magnesium, zinc, and B vitamins. Examples of high fiber grains include:

- Whole grain bread or English muffin

- Sprouted grain bread

- Wheat bran cereal

- Quinoa, barley, bulgur

High Fiber Supplements

Also called functional fiber, high fiber supplements can be an easy way to meet your daily needs. While high fiber supplements may provide similar digestive benefits, they could cause you to miss out on key vitamins, minerals, and phytonutrients that only whole foods can give. The Academy of Nutrition and Dietetics recommends no more than 10 grams of supplemental fiber each day, as too much can have a laxative effect. Before you take supplements, talk to your doctor or pharmacist first to determine if they make sense for your health needs.

Regardless, most nutritionists would agree that best sources of fiber are whole, unprocessed foods. However, if you are choosing a fiber-enriched food, read the label to assure a smart choice. Some foods such as yogurt and cereal are "fiber-fortified," meaning an isolated amount of fiber is added during manufacturing. For example, Fiber One Bran Cereal contains over 10 grams of fiber, an amount that may cause an upset stomach. Additionally, the cereal contains artificial ingredients such as caramel color and sucralose. Lookout for these popular processed foods that are commonly fiber-fortified:

- Yogurt

- Energy bars

- Cereal

- White bread

What other things does fiber do?

Research has shown that a diet rich in fiber is associated with many health benefits, including the following:

1. Lowers cholesterol: Soluble fiber has been shown to lower cholesterol by binding to bile (composed of cholesterol) and taking it out of the body. This may help reduce the risk of heart disease.

2. Better regulates blood sugar levels: A high-fiber meal slows down the digestion of food into the intestines, which may help to keep blood sugars from rising rapidly.

3. Weight control: A high-fiber diet may help keep you fuller longer, which prevents overeating and hunger between meals.

4. May prevent intestinal cancer: Insoluble fiber increases the bulk and speed of food moving through the intestinal tract, which reduces time for harmful substances to build up.

5. Constipation: Constipation can often be relieved by increasing the fiber or roughage in your diet. Fiber works to help regulate bowel movements by pulling water into the colon to produce softer, bulkier stools. This action helps to promote better regularity.

Dangers and Side Effects

You should strive to introduce fiber to your diet slowly. It may take some time for your intestines to get up to speed with the increased digestion of the substance. Eating more fiber than your body can currently handle may cause gas, cramps, and bloating. Ramping up the diet by adding five grams per day may help reduce the gas that commonly accompanies new high-fiber programs. Remember to make healthy choices involving nutrition along with fiber intake. High-fiber food choices may help alleviate the symptoms of many common health issues. Some doctors recommend a specialized high-fiber diet plan for diverticulitis sufferers, for example, but those suffering from health problems should still contact a doctor before making changes to follow instructions found in any diet guide.

How much fiber should I eat?

The Academy of Nutrition and Dietetics recommends consuming about 25-35 grams of total fiber per day, with 10-15 grams from soluble fiber or 14g of fiber per 1,000 calories. This can be accomplished by choosing 6 ounces of grains (3 or more ounces from whole grains),

2½ cups of vegetables, and 2 cups of fruit per day (based on a 2,000 calorie/day pattern). However, as we age, fiber requirements decrease. For those over the age of 70, the recommendation for women is 21 grams and for men 30 grams of total fiber per day.

Note: Eating a high-fiber diet may interfere with the absorption and effectiveness of some medications. Speak to your doctor about which medications to take with caution and when to take them. Fiber also binds with certain nutrients and carries them out of the body. To avoid this, aim for the recommended 20-35 grams of fiber per day. When eating a high-fiber diet, be sure to drink at least eight glasses of fluid each day.

Tips for increasing dietary fiber in your diet:

• Add fiber to your diet slowly. Too much fiber all at once may cause cramping, bloating, and constipation.

• When adding fiber to your diet, be sure to drink adequate fluids (at least 64 ounces or 8 cups per day) to prevent constipation.

• Choose products that have a whole grain listed as the first ingredient, not enriched flour. Whole wheat flour is a whole grain--wheat flour is not.

• Choose whole grain bread with 2-4 grams of dietary fiber per slice.

• Choose cereals with at least 5 grams of dietary fiber per serving.

• Choose raw fruits and vegetables in place of juice, and eat the skins.

- Try alternative fiber choices such as whole buckwheat, whole wheat couscous, quinoa, bulgur, wheat germ, chia seeds, hemp seeds, lentil pasta, and edamame pasta.

- Popcorn is a whole grain. Serve it low-fat without butter for a healthier snack choice.

- Sprinkle bran in soups, cereals, baked products, spaghetti sauce, ground meat, and casseroles. Bran also mixes well with orange juice.

- Use dried peas, beans, and legumes in main dishes, salads, or side dishes such as rice or pasta.

- Add dried fruit to yogurt, cereal, rice, and muffins.

- Try brown rice and whole grain pastas.

CHAPTER TWO

High-Fiber Diet Meal Plan

A standard high-fiber meal plan is rich in fruits and vegetables. Whole grains and beans deliver much of the fiber content for each meal, allowing you to enjoy many different food options while still maintaining your high-fiber diet. Other food choices for a standard meal plan include:

- Broccoli

- Green peas

- Artichokes

These foods are packed with extra nutrition as well as fiber, giving you the vitamins and minerals you need to stay healthy and enjoy an active lifestyle. Brown rice is preferred over standard white varieties, as it contains many more nutrients. Similarly, bran is often separated from whole grains, but it is actually the outer hull of these grains and contains many nutrients that processed varieties lack. Berries are rich in both fiber and antioxidants, making them a great choice for most meal plans. High-fiber meals should deliver around thirty-five grams of fiber per day.

Diet Plan If You Want Weight Loss

Berries and fruits are not usually the best choice when you are following a high-fiber plan for weight loss, however. While they may contain exceptional levels of nutrition and fiber, they are also rich in sugars and high in calories. Instead of making half of your plate consist of both fruits and vegetables, as you would with most standard high-fiber plans, try eating only a single serving or two of fruit per day and adding more leafy vegetables or beans to your meals. These foods are also rich in fiber but much lower in total caloric count. Alcohol and additional sugars should be avoided entirely, as they add no additional fiber and deliver increased calories with little to no nutritional benefit. They can also lead to blood-sugar fluctuations.

Diet Plan for Adding Muscle Mass

Bodybuilders and those looking to add muscle mass as well as trim away body fat may need a combination high-protein and high-fiber plan. Most beans offer a decent source of fiber and protein, making them a staple for plans of this type. Meals should employ a combination of:

- Lean meats

- Beans

- Nuts

- Seeds

All of these food types have extra protein that can help accelerate muscle growth while helping to prevent the low caloric intake of weight-loss diets from causing the body to break down existing muscle tissue. Other great choices for those looking to mix protein and fiber for enhanced muscle growth include:

- Peas

- Complex breads

- Cereals

As with other diet varieties, increased food intake should be met with increased physical activity for best results.

A Typical High-Fiber Week

Those on high-fiber plans are likely to enjoy a variety of different foods throughout the week. Breakfast may start with a rich whole-grain muffin, cup of vegetable juice, and eggs or a lean meat option along with a side of vegetables. Lunch is likely to be made of at least half steamed or raw vegetables and fruits along with a quarter portion of meat and as a quarter portion of beans, nuts, or a similar high-fiber food. Dinner may focus equally as heavily on vegetables and high-fiber options, with beans including black-eyed peas and lima or pinto varieties taking center stage. As with most meals, a combination of fruits and vegetables should make up about half of dinner to introduce extra fiber and help keep calories in check.

Great Food Choices

While there are many great food choices for this plan, a few stand out due to their exceptional levels of nutrition and fiber. Sprinkle high-fiber garnitures onto your foods to increase fiber intake, these include:

• Wheat germ

• Wheat bran

• Oat bran

Similarly, whole-grain breads are a great choice when it comes time to make toast at breakfast or prepare sandwiches for lunch. Sweet potatoes, spinach, and most leafy greens contain excellent nutrition and high fiber levels. For a light snack, try air-popped popcorn, which contains up to four grams of fiber for each popped cup. Almonds and peanuts are also great snack foods that may be easily incorporated in to different meals.

Recipe for All Plans

Whether your meal plan calls for additional veggies, meats, or even more sources of fiber, this simple recipe is a great choice. You can also easily modify it to create multiple meals. Lightly toast two pieces of whole-grain bread and serve them along with steamed beans and a meat of your choice. Grilled meat offers a healthy alternative to fried varieties. Add leafy green vegetables for added nutrition; available choices include:

- Spinach

- Kale

- Broccoli

Finish the meal with a low-calorie and low-caffeine beverage. Consider creating parfaits made by mixing five parts yogurt to one part fiber-rich berries and sprinkle with bran for a tasty and healthy dessert.

Here are a couple of recipes you could try:

Spicy Skillet Chicken
Ingredients

- 1 to 2 tea spoons chili powder

- ½ tea spoon salt

- ¼ tea spoon pepper

- 4 boneless skinless chicken breasts (about 1 1/4 lb)

- 1 table spoon vegetable oil

- 1 can (15 oz) Progresso™ black beans, drained, rinsed

- 1 can (11 oz) whole kernel corn with red and green peppers, undrained

- 1/3 cup Old El Paso Thick 'n Chunky salsa

- 2 cups hot cooked rice

Steps

1. In small bowl, mix chili powder, salt and pepper; sprinkle evenly over both sides of chicken breasts.

2. In 10-inch nonstick skillet, heat oil over medium heat. Add chicken; cook 8 to 10 minutes, turning once, until juice of chicken is clear when center of thickest part is cut (170°F).

3. Stir in beans, corn and salsa. Heat to boiling. Reduce heat. Cover and simmer 3 to 5 minutes or until vegetables are hot. Serve with rice.

Slow-Cooker Black Beans and Rice

Traditional black beans and rice is made slow cooker easy without sacrificing the spices and seasoning this dish is famous for.

Ingredients

- 1 lb dried black beans (2 cups), sorted, rinsed
- 1 large onion, chopped (1 cup)
- 1 large bell pepper, chopped (1 1/2 cups)
- 5 cloves garlic, finely chopped
- 2 dried bay leaves
- 1 can (14.5 oz) Muir Glen™ organic diced tomatoes, undrained
- 5 cups water
- 2 table spoons olive or vegetable oil
- 4 tea spoons ground cumin

- 2 tea spoons finely chopped jalapeño chilies

- 1 tea spoon salt

- 3 cups hot cooked rice

Steps

1. In 3 1/2- to 6-quart slow cooker, mix all Ingredients except rice.

2. Cover; cook on High heat setting 6 to 8 hours.

3. Remove bay leaves. Serve beans over rice. Note: This recipe was tested in slow cookers with heating elements in the side and bottom of the cooker, not in cookers that stand only on a heated base. For slow cookers with just a heated base, follow the manufacturer's directions for layering Ingredients and choosing a temperature.

Lemon Cake Pops

This quick dessert hack gives you glazed lemon cake pops in a matter of minutes.

Ingredients

- 1 Fiber One™ 90 calorie lemon bar
- 2 tablespoons powdered sugar
- ½ teaspoon water
- Zest from 1 lemon
- 1 cake pop stick

Steps

1. Mix a glaze of water and powdered sugar.
2. Roll that tangy lemon bar into a uniform ball.
3. Dip the ball into the glaze.
4. Sprinkle your pop with lemon zest.

5. Pop it on the stick and enjoy.

Pasta and Bean Skillet

Saddle up your family for this easy pasta and bean skillet. It has a great chili taste that's worth hitting the trail for.

Ingredients

- 1 cup Old El Paso™ salsa (any variety)

- 2/3 cup uncooked elbow macaroni (2 ounces)

- ¾ cup water

- 2 teaspoons chili powder

- 2 cups Progresso™ red kidney beans (from 19-oz can), drained, rinsed

- 1 can (8 ounces) tomato sauce

- ½ cup shredded Cheddar cheese (2 ounces)

Steps

1. Heat all Ingredients except cheese to boiling in 10-inch nonstick skillet; reduce heat.

2. Cover and simmer about 15 minutes, stirring frequently, until macaroni is tender. Sprinkle with cheese.

Mocha Coffee Frappé

Blend a chocolaty brownie with coffee, frozen yogurt and chocolate syrup for an indulgent afternoon treat or dessert.

Ingredients

- 1 Fiber One™ 90 Calorie chocolate fudge brownies, chopped into chunks

- ½ cup sugar-free frozen yogurt

- ¼ cup prepared strong coffee, cold

- 3 tablespoons sugar-free chocolate syrup (or to taste)

- ½ cup ice cubes

Steps

1. Combine the Ingredients in your blender and blend until smooth — that means no ice chunks.

Steamed Chinese Vegetables with Brown Rice

Lots of veggies, high-fiber brown rice and a healthful cooking method make this recipe a winner.

Ingredients

- 1 Japanese or regular eggplant, 1 1/2 pounds, cut into 2x1/2-inch strips (3 cups)

- 1 medium red bell pepper, cut into julienne strips (1 1/2 cups)

- 1 large carrot, cut into julienne strips (1 cup)
- 1 cup sliced bok choy stems and leaves
- 1 medium onion, thinly sliced
- ½ pound snow (Chinese) pea pods (2 cups)
- 2 tablespoons soy sauce
- 1 tablespoon creamy peanut butter
- 1 tablespoon hoisin sauce
- 1 teaspoon grated gingerroot
- 1 clove garlic, finely chopped
- 2 cups hot cooked brown rice

Steps

1. Place steamer basket in 1/2 inch water in saucepan or skillet (water should not touch bottom of basket). Place eggplant, bell pepper,

carrot, bok choy and onion in steamer basket. Cover tightly and heat to boiling; reduce heat to medium-low. Steam 5 to 8 minutes, adding pea pods for the last minute of steaming, until vegetables are crisp-tender.

2. Beat soy sauce, peanut butter, hoisin sauce, gingerroot and garlic in large bowl with wire whisk until blended. Add vegetables; toss. Serve over rice.

Grilled Barbecued Beef and Bean Burgers

With beefy bean burgers that are ready in less than 30 minutes, you can have your meat and fiber, too.

Ingredients

- ½ lb extra-lean (at least 90%) ground beef

- 1 can (15 to 16 oz) great northern beans, drained, rinsed

- ¼ cup finely crushed saltine crackers (about 7 squares)

- 2 tablespoons barbecue sauce

- ¼ teaspoon pepper

- 1 egg

- Leaf lettuce, if desired

- 5 whole-grain hamburger buns, split

- 5 teaspoons barbecue sauce

- Sliced tomato and sliced onion, if desired

Steps

1. Heat gas or charcoal grill. In large bowl, mix beef, beans, cracker crumbs, 2 tablespoons

barbecue sauce, the pepper and egg. Shape into 5 patties, about 1/2 inch thick.

2. Brush grill rack with vegetable oil. Place patties on grill. Cover grill; cook over medium heat 5 minutes. Turn; cook covered 5 to 6 minutes longer or until meat thermometer inserted in center of patties reads 160°F.

3. Place lettuce and patties on bottom halves of buns. Spread each patty with 1 teaspoon barbecue sauce. Top with tomato and onion. Cover with bun tops.

Red Bean and Rice Cakes
Make a meatless main dish that's high on flavor and fiber. Chili powder, cumin, cayenne and salsa elevate the flavor, while cereal adds crunch and fiber.

Ingredients

- ½ cup uncooked regular long-grain white rice
- 1 cup water
- 1 cup Fiber One™ original bran cereal
- 2 cans (15 oz each) Progresso™ dark red kidney beans, drained, rinsed
- 1 small onion, finely chopped (1/4 cup)
- ¼ cup diced green bell pepper
- 1 egg or 2 egg whites, beaten
- 1 tablespoon chili powder
- 1 teaspoon ground cumin
- ¼ teaspoon ground red pepper (cayenne)
- Salad greens, if desired
- ½ cup Old El Paso Thick 'n Chunky salsa

Steps

1. Cook rice in water as directed on package. Meanwhile, place cereal in resealable food-storage plastic bag; seal bag and crush with rolling pin or meat mallet (or crush in food processor).

2. In large bowl, place beans; mash with potato masher or fork. Stir in onion, bell pepper, cooked rice, egg, chili powder, cumin, red pepper and 2 tablespoons of the cereal. Shape into 8 patties; coat patties completely with remaining cereal.

3. Spray 10-inch skillet with cooking spray. Cook 4 patties in skillet over medium heat about 10 minutes, turning once, until brown. Remove patties from skillet. Cover and keep warm while cooking remaining patties.

4. Serve patties on salad greens; top with salsa.

Lentil-Vegetable Soup

Wholesome and hot--just the right soup for a chilly day.

Ingredients

- 1 large onion, chopped (1 cup)
- 2 teaspoons chili powder
- 1 teaspoon salt
- 1 teaspoon ground cumin
- 2 cloves garlic, finely chopped
- 1 can (6 oz) spicy tomato juice
- 3cups water
- 1 cup (8 oz) dried lentils, sorted, rinsed
- 2 cups Muir Glen™ organic diced tomatoes (from 28-oz can), undrained
- 1 can (4.5 oz) Old El Paso™ chopped green chiles, undrained

- 1 cup fresh or frozen whole kernel corn

- 2 small zucchini, cut into julienne strips (2 cups)

Steps

1. In 3-quart saucepan, heat onion, chili powder, salt, cumin, garlic and tomato juice to boiling. Reduce heat; cover and simmer 5 minutes.

2. Stir in water, lentils, tomatoes and chiles. Heat to boiling. Reduce heat; cover and simmer 20 minutes.

3. Stir in corn. Cover; simmer 10 minutes. Stir in zucchini. Cover; simmer about 5 minutes or until lentils and zucchini are tender.

Chocolate Fudge Brownie Berry Sundae

Ingredients

- 1 Fiber One 90 Calorie chocolate fudge brownie
- 1 tbsp. raspberry sorbet
- 6 fresh raspberries

Steps

1. Place brownie in individual serving bowl. Spoon sorbet on top of brownie. Dot sorbet with fresh raspberries.

Mexican Chocolate Cream Pie

Cinnamon coffee cake atop a bed of creamy chocolate-cinnamon mixture makes for a quick and tasty treat.

Ingredients

- 1 Fiber One™ 90 calorie cinnamon coffee cake
- 1/3 cup sugar-free fat-free instant chocolate pudding, fully prepared
- 1/4 cup plain, nonfat greek yogurt
- 1/8 teaspoon ground cinnamon
- 3 tablespoons Cool Whip fat-free frozen whipped topping, thawed

Steps

1. Whisk together the pudding, yogurt and cinnamon and spoon the mixture over the bar

2. Stick it in the fridge for 30 minutes

3. Take it out and add a dollop of whipped cream

Lemon Strawberry Shortcake Trifle

Layer lemon bar crumbles with fresh strawberries and a Greek yogurt-lemon pudding mix for a healthier trifle twist.

Ingredients

- 1 Fiber One™ 90 calorie lemon bar, crumbled
- 1/3 cup sugar-free, fat-free instant lemon pudding, fully prepared
- 1/3 cup nonfat Greek yogurt
- 1/3 cup fresh strawberries, sliced

Steps

1. Break apart a lemon bar and some strawberries and swirl together Greek yogurt with a little lemon pudding. Create two layers of each and you've got yourself a light and sweet treat.

Chicken and Northern Beans White Chili

Chili is one of our go-to winter dishes but there comes a time, about halfway through the season, when we tire of all our favorite cold weather recipes. If you know the feeling, we suggest this recipe as an antidote! It's got all the heartiness of your standard bowl o' .

Ingredients

- ¼ cup butter or margarine

- 1 large onion, chopped (1 cup)

- 1 garlic clove, finely chopped

- 4 cups 1/2-inch cubes cooked chicken or turkey

- 3 cups Progresso chicken broth (from 32-oz carton)

- 2 table spoons chopped fresh cilantro

- 1 table spoon dried basil leaves

- 2 tea spoons ground red chilies or Chili powder

- ¼ tea spoon ground cloves

- 2 cans (15 to 16 oz each) great northern beans, undrained

- 1 medium tomato, chopped (3/4 cup)

- Blue or yellow corn tortilla chips

Steps

1. Melt butter in 4-quart Dutch oven over medium heat. Cook onion and garlic in butter, stirring occasionally until onion is tender.

2. Stir in remaining Ingredients except tomato and tortilla chips. Heat to boiling; reduce heat. Cover and simmer 1 hour, stirring occasionally. Serve with tomato and tortilla chips.

Vegetarian Vegetable and Bean Chili

When it feels like your pantry is bare, but you've got a hungry family to feed, this recipe is a surefire solution. Made with canned beans, frozen vegetables and a couple of standard Ingredients, it'll make you feel like you've made something out of nothing.

Ingredients

- 1 table spoon olive or vegetable oil

- 2 medium onions, coarsely chopped (1 cup)

- 2 teaspoons finely chopped garlic

- 2 cups frozen corn

- 1 bag (1 lb) frozen broccoli, carrots and cauliflower

- 1 can (19 oz) Progresso™ red kidney beans, drained, rinsed

- 1 can (15 oz) Progresso™ chickpeas (garbanzo beans), drained, rinsed

- 2 cans (14.5 oz each) diced tomatoes with green chiles, undrained

- 1 can (8 oz) tomato sauce

- 2 table spoons chili powder

- 3 tea spoons ground cumin

- 3/4 tea spoon salt

- 1/8 tea spoon ground red pepper (cayenne)

Steps

1. In 4 1/2- to 5-quart Dutch oven, heat oil over medium-high heat. Add onions and garlic; cook 4 to 5 minutes, stirring frequently, until onions are softened.

2. Stir in remaining Ingredients. Heat to boiling. Reduce heat to medium-low. Cover; cook 15 to 20 minutes, stirring occasionally, until chili is hot and vegetables are crisp-tender.

Blueberry Cinnamon Coffeecake

This warm coffee cake with a generous serving of blueberries is a great way to jump-start your mornings.

Ingredients

- 1 Fiber One™ 90 Calorie Cinnamon Coffee Cake
- 1 teaspoon blueberry preserves
- 1 tablespoon fresh blueberries (about 8 or 9)
- 1 teaspoon sliced almonds

Steps

1. On a heatproof dish, warm coffee cake in the microwave for 10 to 15 seconds. Top with the preserves, fresh blueberries and almonds.

Oatmeal Raisin Cookie Ice Cream Sandwich

Sandwich frozen yogurt and dark chocolate chips in between two oatmeal-raisin cookies for a tasty twist on ice cream sandwiches.

Ingredients

- 1 Fiber One™ 120 calorie oatmeal raisin cookie

- ¼ cup sugar-free vanilla frozen yogurt

- ½ tablespoon mini dark chocolate chips

Steps

1. Cut your cookie in half and scoop the ice cream on top of one half. Top it with the other half of your cookie and roll the exposed ice cream in chocolate chips.

Dutch Oven Black Bean Soup

The interesting blend of spices in this soup will remind you of the traditional Cuban meal of black beans and rice.

Ingredients

- 2 2/3 cups dried black beans (1 lb)

- 2 table spoons vegetable oil

- 1 large onion, chopped (1 cup)

- 3 cloves garlic, finely chopped

- 3 cups Progresso™ beef flavored broth (from 32-oz carton) or vegetable broth

- 3 cups water

- ¼ cup dark rum or apple cider

- 1 tea spoon liquid smoke

- 1 ½ tea spoons ground cumin

- 1 ½ tea spoons dried oregano leaves

- 1 medium green bell pepper, chopped (1 cup)

- 1 large tomato, chopped (1 cup)

Steps

1. Place beans in Dutch oven; add enough cold water to cover beans. Heat to boiling. Boil uncovered 2 minutes. Remove from heat; cover and let stand 1 hour. Drain and reserve beans.

2. In same Dutch oven, heat oil over medium heat. Add onion and garlic; cook, stirring occasionally, until onion is tender.

3. Stir in remaining Ingredients. Heat to boiling. Boil 2 minutes. Reduce heat to low; cover and simmer about 2 hours or until beans are tender.

4. Carefully pour soup into blender. Cover; blend until almost smooth.

Mini Peanut Butter Brownie Cupcake

Top a Fiber One™ 90 calorie chocolate peanut butter brownie with hazelnut spread and pecans for a treat ready in five minutes!

Ingredients

- 1 Fiber One™ 90 calorie chocolate peanut butter brownie

- 1 tablespoon hazelnut spread

- 1 pecan

- Pinch sea salt

Steps

1. Press a brownie into a mini cupcake pan to mold it into the shape of a cupcake.

2. To get it out of the pan, use a spoon to loosen one side of the brownie, then flip the pan over and let gravity do the rest.

3. Frost your cupcake with hazelnut spread and top it with your pecan and sea salt.

Frozen Yogurt Cookie Sundae

Ingredients

- 1 Fiber One™ 90 calorie chocolate chip cookie bar

- 1 tbsp. vanilla fat-free frozen yogurt, slightly softened

- ½ tsp. M&M's® minis chocolate candies

- ½ tsp. light chocolate-flavor syrup

Steps

1. Place cookie in serving bowl. Spoon frozen yogurt on top; sprinkle with candies. Drizzle with chocolate syrup.

Upside Down Lemon Cream Pie

Try this tasty dessert hack using a Fiber One™ 90 calorie lemon bar and a Greek yogurt-lemon pudding topping.

Ingredients

- 1 Fiber One™ 90 calorie lemon bar

- 1/3 cup sugar-free, fat-free instant lemon pudding, prepared

- 1/3 cup plain, nonfat Greek yogurt

- 1 tablespoon Cool Whip fat-free frozen whipped topping, thawed

- 1 tablespoon unsweetened shredded coconut

Steps

1. Top off a lemon bar with Greek yogurt and lemon pudding mixture and stick it in the fridge for 30 minutes. Add a dollop of whipped cream, a lemon wedge and coconut flakes and enjoy!

Mango Lemon Leche

This fruity snack topped with fresh mangos is perfect for any time of day.

Ingredients

- 1 Fiber One™ 90 calorie lemon bar

- 2 tablespoons of fat-free plain kefir

- 1 tablespoon of mango sauce (1/3 mango and 1 tablespoon water)

- 2 fresh mango spheres

Steps

1. Pour kefir and homemade mango sauce in a shallow bowl, place lemon bar on top and garnish with two mango spheres.

Chocolate and Pear Coffee Cake

Top coffee cake with chocolate pudding drizzle and chopped pecans for a sweet snack.

Ingredients

- 1 Fiber One™ 90 calorie cinnamon coffee cake

- 1 tablespoon of fat-free chocolate pudding snack

- ½ fresh Bosc pear

Steps

1. Place a Fiber One Cinnamon Coffee Cake on a plate

2. Top with chopped pears and drizzle with chocolate pudding.

Cinnamon and Lime Chicken Fajitas

Spicy, addictive, easy to make - you can't stop eating these! The potato puts it over the top! Well worth the time. Serve with salsa, cheese, cilantro, and sour cream. Great with beans and rice!

Ingredients

- 4 boneless, skinless chicken breast halves

- 1 tablespoon ground cinnamon

- 1 tablespoon salt and pepper to taste

- 2 large baking potatoes, peeled and cubed

- ¼ cup canola oil

- 1 large yellow onion, chopped

- 1 large clove garlic, peeled and minced

- 1 tablespoon chopped jalapeno peppers

- 1 lime, juiced

- 12 (6 inch) corn tortillas, warmed

Steps

1. Preheat oven to 400 degrees F (200 degrees C).

2. Place potatoes in a shallow baking dish. Drizzle with about 1/2 the oil, and season with salt. Bake 30 to 40 minutes in the preheated oven, until tender.

3. Meanwhile, season chicken with cinnamon, salt, and pepper. Arrange in a separate baking

dish, and bake 30 minutes in the preheated oven, until no longer pink and juices run clear. Cool and shred.

4. Heat remaining oil in a skillet over medium heat, and saute onion and garlic until tender. Mix in shredded chicken, jalapeno, and lime juice. Cook until heated through.

5. Serve the chicken and potatoes in warmed tortillas.

Fiery Fish Tacos with Crunchy Corn Salsa

Spicy grilled fish are cooled down with a fresh crunchy veggie salsa featuring fresh corn. Your guests will swim back for seconds!

Ingredients

- 2 cups cooked corn kernels

- 1/2 cup diced red onion
- 1 cup peeled, diced jicama
- 1/2 cup diced red bell pepper
- 1 cup fresh cilantro leaves, chopped
- 1 lime, juiced and zested
- 2 table spoons cayenne pepper, or to taste
- 1 table spoon ground black pepper
- 2 table spoons salt, or to taste
- 6 (4 ounce) fillets tilapia
- 2 tablespoons olive oil
- 12 corn tortillas, warmed
- 2 table spoons sour cream, or to taste

Steps

1. Preheat grill for high heat.

2. In a medium bowl, mix together corn, red onion, jicama, red bell pepper, and cilantro. Stir in lime juice and zest.

3. In a small bowl, combine cayenne pepper, ground black pepper, and salt.

4. Brush each fillet with olive oil, and sprinkle with spices to taste.

5. Arrange fillets on grill grate, and cook for 3 minutes per side. For each fiery fish taco, top two corn tortillas with fish, sour cream, and corn salsa.

Quinoa and Black Beans

Very flavorful alternative to black beans and rice. Quinoa is a nutty grain from South America.

Ingredients

- 1 tea spoon vegetable oil
- 1 onion, chopped
- 3 cloves garlic, chopped
- ¾ cup quinoa
- 1 ½ cups vegetable broth
- 1 tea spoon ground cumin
- ¼ tea spoon cayenne pepper
- salt and ground black pepper to taste
- 1 cup frozen corn kernels

- 2 (15 ounce) cans black beans, rinsed and drained

- ½ cup chopped fresh cilantro

Steps

1. Heat oil in a saucepan over medium heat; cook and stir onion and garlic until lightly browned, about 10 minutes.

2. Mix quinoa into onion mixture and cover with vegetable broth; season with cumin, cayenne pepper, salt, and pepper. Bring the mixture to a boil. Cover, reduce heat, and simmer until quinoa is tender and broth is absorbed, about 20 minutes.

3. Stir frozen corn into the saucepan, and continue to simmer until heated through, about 5 minutes; mix in the black beans and cilantro.

Simple Baked Beans

This baked bean recipe uses canned beans instead of the dry type so it is quick and easy to prepare.

Ingredients

- 2 (16 ounce) cans baked beans with pork
- ¼ cup molasses
- ¼ cup chopped onions
- 4 tablespoons brown sugar
- 1 tablespoon prepared mustard
- 2 tablespoons ketchup
- 2 slices bacon, chopped

Steps

1. Preheat oven to 350 degrees F (175 degrees C).

2. Mix baked beans with pork, molasses, onions, brown sugar and ketchup together and put in a greased casserole dish. Top with bacon, cover and bake for 3 hours or until thick.

Wendy's Quick Pasta and Lentils

Hearty pasta and lentil dish. Sure to warm you down to your toes! Serve with Parmesan and crusty bread.

Ingredients

- 1 onion, chopped

- 3 cloves garlic, minced

- 2 tablespoons olive oil

- 1 (19 ounce) can lentil soup
- 1 cup crushed tomatoes
- 1 (10 ounce) package frozen chopped spinach
- 1 (16 ounce) package ditalini pasta salt to taste
- ground black pepper to taste
- 1 pinch crushed red pepper
- 2 tablespoons grated Parmesan cheese

Steps

1. Brown onion and garlic in oil over medium heat. Stir in lentil soup and tomatoes. Bring to boil. Stir in spinach and spices. Simmer.

2. Meanwhile, cook pasta in a large pot of boiling salted water until almost done. Drain. Mix pasta into lentil sauce. Cover, and keep warm for 20 minutes. Serve with Parmesan cheese.

Whole Wheat Pasta

Fresh, healthy and very delish...

Ingredients

- 1 1/2 cups all-purpose flour

- 1 1/2 cups whole wheat flour

- 1/2 teaspoon sea salt

- 4 eggs

- 2 tea spoons olive oil

Steps

1. Stir together the all-purpose flour, whole wheat flour and salt in a medium bowl, or on a clean board. Make a hollow in the center, and pour in the olive oil. Break eggs into it one at a time, while mixing quickly with a fork until the dough is wet enough to come together. Knead on a lightly floured surface until the dough is stiff

and elastic. Cover, and let stand for 30 minutes to relax.

2. Roll out dough by hand with a rolling pin, or use a pasta machine to achieve the desired thickness of noodles. Cut into desired width and shapes. Allow the pasta to air dry for at least 15 minutes to avoid having it clump together.

To cook fresh pasta:

Bring a large pot of lightly salted water to a boil. Add the pasta, and cook for 2 to 3 minutes. Fresh pasta cooks very quickly. It will float to the surface when fully cooked. Drain, and use as desired.

Chinese Chicken Salad III
Ingredients

- 3 table spoons hoisin sauce

- 2 table spoons peanut butter

- 2 tea spoons brown sugar

- ¾ tea spoon hot chile paste

- 1 teaspoon grated fresh ginger

- 3 tablespoons rice wine vinegar

- 1 tablespoon sesame oil

- 1 pound skinless, boneless chicken breast halves

- 16 (3.5 inch square) wonton wrappers, shredded

- 4 cups romaine lettuce - torn, washed and dried

- 2 cups shredded carrots

- 1 bunch green onions, chopped

- ¼ cup chopped fresh cilantro

Steps

1. To prepare the dressing, whisk together the hoisin sauce, peanut butter, brown sugar, chili paste, ginger, vinegar, and sesame oil.

2. Grill or broil the chicken breasts until cooked, about 10 minutes. An instant-read thermometer inserted into the center should read 165 degrees F (74 degrees C). Cool and slice.

3. Preheat oven to 350 degrees F (175 C). Spray a large shallow pan with nonstick vegetable spray; arrange shredded wontons in a single layer and bake until golden brown, about 20 minutes. Cool.

4. In a large bowl, combine the chicken, wontons, lettuce, carrots, green onions and cilantro. Toss with dressing and serve.

Irish Chicken and Dumplings

Ingredients

- 2 (10.75 ounce) cans condensed cream of chicken soup

- 3 cups water

- 1 cup chopped celery

- 2 onions, quartered

- 1 tea spoon salt

- ½ tea spoon poultry seasoning

- ½ tea spoon ground black pepper

- 4 skinless, boneless chicken breast halves

- 5 carrots, sliced

- 1 (10 ounce) package frozen green peas

- 4 medium (2-1/4" to 3" dia, raw)s potatoes, quartered

- 3 cups baking mix

- 1 ⅓ cups milk

Steps

1. In large, heavy pot, combine soup, water, chicken, celery, onion, salt, poultry seasoning, and pepper. Cover and cook over low heat about 1 1/2 hours.

2. Add potatoes and carrots; cover and cook another 30 minutes.

3. Remove chicken from pot, shred it, and return to pot. Add peas and cook only 5 minutes longer.

4. Add dumplings. To make dumplings: Mix baking mix and milk until a soft dough forms. Drop by tablespoonfuls onto BOILING stew. Simmer covered for 10 minutes, then uncover and simmer an additional 10 minutes.

Vegetarian Chickpea Sandwich Filling

Serve this tasty sandwich spread on crusty whole grain rolls or pita bread, with lettuce and tomato. Other raw, chopped vegetables can be substituted for the celery. Your favorite salad dressing can be substituted for the mayo.

Ingredients

- 1 (19 ounce) can garbanzo beans, drained and rinsed

- 1 stalk celery, chopped

- 1/2 onion, chopped

- 1 tablespoon mayonnaise

- 1 tablespoon lemon juice

- 1 teaspoon dried dill weedsalt and pepper to taste

Steps

1. Drain and rinse chickpeas. Pour chickpeas into a medium size mixing bowl and mash with a fork. Mix in celery, onion, mayonnaise (to taste), lemon juice, dill, salt and pepper to taste.

Greek Chicken Pasta

This pasta dish incorporates some of the flavors of Greece. It makes a wonderfully complete and satisfying meal. For extra flavor, toss in a few kalamata olives. Use whatever pasta you have or prefer.

Ingredients

- 1 (16 ounce) package linguine pasta

- ½ cup chopped red onion

- 1 tablespoon olive oil

- 2 cloves garlic, crushed

- 1 pound skinless, boneless chicken breast meat - cut into bite-size pieces

- 1 (14 ounce) can marinated artichoke hearts, drained and chopped

- 1 large tomato, chopped

- ½ cup crumbled feta cheese

- 3 tablespoons chopped fresh parsley

- 2 tablespoons lemon juice

- 2 teaspoons dried oregano

- salt and pepper to taste

- 2 lemons, wedged, for garnish

Steps

1. Bring a large pot of lightly salted water to a boil. Cook pasta in boiling water until tender yet firm to the bit, 8 to 10 minutes; drain.

2. Heat olive oil in a large skillet over medium-high heat. Add onion and garlic; saute until fragrant, about 2 minutes. Stir in the chicken and cook, stirring occasionally, until chicken is no longer pink in the center and the juices run clear, about 5 to 6 minutes.

3. Reduce heat to medium-low; add artichoke hearts, tomato, feta cheese, parsley, lemon juice, oregano, and cooked pasta. Cook and stir until heated through, about 2 to 3 minutes. Remove from heat, season with salt and pepper, and garnish with lemon wedges.

Red Lentil Curry

This is a rich and hearty lentil curry, great as a main meal rather than as a side dish like the more traditional Indian dhal. Don't let the ingredient list faze you, this really is an easy dish to make. This dish is great served with basmati rice.

Ingredients

- 2 cups red lentils

- 1 large onion, diced

- 1 table spoon vegetable oil

- 2 table spoons curry paste

- 1 table spoon curry powder

- 1 tea spoon ground turmeric

- 1 tea spoon ground cumin

- 1 tea spoon chili powder
- 1 tea spoon salt
- 1 tea spoon white sugar
- 1 tea spoon minced garlic
- 1 tea spoon minced fresh ginger
- 1 (14.25 ounce) can tomato puree

Steps

1. Wash the lentils in cold water until the water runs clear. Put lentils in a pot with enough water to cover; bring to a boil, place a cover on the pot, reduce heat to medium-low, and simmer, adding water during cooking as needed to keep covered, until tender, 15 to 20 minutes. Drain.

2. Heat vegetable oil in a large skillet over medium heat; cook and stir onions in hot oil until caramelized, about 20 minutes.

3. Mix curry paste, curry powder, turmeric, cumin, chili powder, salt, sugar, garlic, and ginger together in a large bowl; stir into the onions. Increase heat to high and cook, stirring constantly, until fragrant, 1 to 2 minutes.

4. Stir in the tomato puree, remove from heat and stir into the lentils.

Chickpea Curry

We usually recommend preparing the beans at home, but using canned chickpeas allows for a fast, convenient dish.

Ingredients

2 cloves garlic, minced

2 tea spoons fresh ginger root, finely chopped

6 whole cloves

2 (2 inch) sticks cinnamon, crushed

1 tea spoon ground cumin

1 tea spoon ground coriander salt

1 tea spoon cayenne pepper

1 tea spoon ground turmeric

2 (15 ounce) cans garbanzo beans

1 cup chopped fresh cilantro

Steps

1. Heat oil in a large frying pan over medium heat, and fry onions until tender.

2. Stir in garlic, ginger, cloves, cinnamon, cumin, coriander, salt, cayenne, and turmeric. Cook for 1

minute over medium heat, stirring constantly. Mix in garbanzo beans and their liquid. Continue to cook and stir until all ingredients are well blended and heated through. Remove from heat. Stir in cilantro just before serving, reserving 1 tablespoon for garnish.

Southwest Chicken

Chicken breasts with black beans, corn, chile peppers, tomatoes. Low-fat, easy and quick. Serve over hot cooked rice if desired.

Ingredients

- 1 tablespoon vegetable oil

- 4 skinless, boneless chicken breast halves

- 1 (10 ounce) can diced tomatoes with green chile peppers

- 1 (15 ounce) can black beans, rinsed and drained

- 1 (8.75 ounce) can whole kernel corn, drained

- 1 pinch ground cumin

Steps

1. In a large skillet, heat oil over medium high heat. Brown chicken breasts on both sides. Add tomatoes with green chile peppers, beans and corn. Reduce heat and let simmer for 25 to 30 minutes or until chicken is cooked through and juices run clear. Add a dash of cumin and serve.

Slow Cooker Chicken Cacciatore

Easy slow cooker chicken cacciatore. Serve over angel hair pasta. 'Cacciatore' is Italian for 'hunter', and this American-Italian term refers to food prepared 'hunter style,' with mushrooms and onions. Avanti!

Ingredients

- 6 skinless, boneless chicken breast halves
- 1 (28 ounce) jar spaghetti sauce
- 2 green bell pepper, seeded and cubed
- 8 ounces fresh mushrooms, sliced
- 1 onion, finely diced
- 2 tablespoons minced garlic

Steps

1. Put the chicken in the slow cooker. Top with the spaghetti sauce, green bell peppers, mushrooms, onion, and garlic.

2. Cover, and cook on Low for 7 to 9 hours.

Black Beans and Rice

Ingredients

1 tea spoon olive oil

1 onion, chopped

2 cloves garlic, minced

3/4 cup uncooked white rice

1 1/2 cups low sodium, low fat vegetable broth

1 tea spoon ground cumin

1/4 tea spoon cayenne pepper

3 1/2 cups canned black beans, drained

Steps

1. In a stockpot over medium-high heat, heat the oil. Add the onion and garlic and saute for 4 minutes. Add the rice and saute for 2 minutes.

2. Add the vegetable broth, bring to a boil, cover and lower the heat and cook for 20 minutes. Add the spices and black beans.

Easy Red Beans and Rice
Ingredients

- 2 cups water

- 1 cup uncooked rice

- 1 (16 ounce) package turkey kielbasa, cut diagonally into 1/4 inch slices

- 1 onion, chopped

- 1 green bell pepper, chopped

- Tri Colored Peppers Red, Yellow & Orange Bell Peppers

- 1 clove chopped garlic

- 2 (15 ounce) cans canned kidney beans, drained

- 1 (16 ounce) can whole peeled tomatoes, chopped

- 1/2 teaspoon dried oregano salt to taste

- 1/2 teaspoon pepper.

Steps

1. In a saucepan, bring water to a boil. Add rice and stir. Reduce heat, cover and simmer for 20 minutes.

2. In a large skillet over low heat, cook sausage for 5 minutes. Stir in onion, green pepper and garlic; saute until tender. Pour in beans and tomatoes with juice. Season with oregano, salt and pepper. Simmer uncovered for 20 minutes. Serve over rice.

Slow Cooker Chicken Marrakesh

Ingredients

- 1 onion, sliced

- 2 cloves garlic, minced

- 2 large carrots, peeled and diced

- 2 large sweet potatoes, peeled and diced

- 1 (15 ounce) can garbanzo beans, drained and rinsed

- 2 pounds skinless, boneless chicken breast halves, cut into 2-inch pieces

- ½ tea spoon ground cumin

- ½ tea spoon ground turmeric

- ¼ tea spoon ground cinnamon

- ½ tea spoon ground black pepper

- 1 tea spoon dried parsley

- 1 tea spoon salt

- 1 (14.5 ounce) can diced tomatoes

Steps

1. Place the onion, garlic, carrots, sweet potatoes, garbanzo beans, and chicken breast pieces into a slow cooker. In a bowl, mix the cumin, turmeric, cinnamon, black pepper, parsley, and salt, and sprinkle over the chicken and vegetables. Pour in the tomatoes, and stir to combine.

2. Cover the cooker, set to High, and cook until the sweet potatoes are tender and the sauce has thickened, 4 to 5 hours.

Garlic Chicken Stir Fry

Ingredients

- 2 table spoons peanut oil

- 6 cloves garlic, minced

- 1 tea spoon grated fresh ginger

- 1 bunch green onions, chopped

- 1 tea spoon salt

- 1 pound boneless skinless chicken breasts, cut into strips

- 2 onions, thinly sliced

- 1 cup sliced cabbage

- 1 red bell pepper, thinly sliced

- 2 cups sugar snap peas

- 1 cup chicken broth

- 2 table spoons soy sauce

- 2 table spoons white sugar

- 2 table spoons cornstarch

Steps

1. Heat peanut oil in a wok or large skillet. When oil begins to smoke, quickly stir in 2 cloves minced garlic, ginger root, green onions and salt. Stir fry until onion becomes translucent, about 2 minutes. Add chicken and stir until opaque, about 3 minutes. Add remaining 4 cloves minced garlic and stir. Add sweet onions, cabbage, bell pepper, peas and 1/2 cup of the broth/water and cover.

2. In a small bowl, mix the remaining 1/2 cup broth/water, soy sauce, sugar and cornstarch. Add sauce mixture to wok/skillet and stir until chicken and vegetables are coated with the

thickened sauce. Serve immediately, over hot rice if desired.

Greek Pasta with Tomatoes and White Beans

An easy, quick, and tasty recipe. The flavors are wonderfully different as they are combined and meld together.

Ingredients

- 2 (14.5 ounce) cans Italian-style diced tomatoes

- 1 (19 ounce) can cannellini beans, drained and rinsed

- 10 ounces fresh spinach, washed and chopped

- 8 ounces penne pasta

- 1/2 cup crumbled feta cheese

Steps

1. Cook the pasta in a large pot of boiling salted water until al dente.

2. Meanwhile, combine tomatoes and beans in a large non-stick skillet. Bring to a boil over medium high heat. Reduce heat, and simmer 10 minutes.

3. Add spinach to the sauce; cook for 2 minutes or until spinach wilts, stirring constantly.

4. Serve sauce over pasta, and sprinkle with feta.

CONCLUSION

Many different studies have highlighted how eating a diet high in fiber can boost your immune system and overall health, and improve how you look and feel.

The most commonly-cited benefit of fiber is its ability to support healthy bowel movements. Dietary fiber bulks up stool to help move waste through your body. Eating a diet rich in high fiber foods can help to prevent constipation, reduce your risk for diverticulitis (inflammation of the intestine), and provide some relief for irritable bowel syndrome (IBS).

An American Journal of Clinical Nutrition study found that fiber acts as natural protective armor against C-reactive protein (CRP), a sign of acute inflammation. When CRP is circulating in the blood, you are more likely to develop diabetes or cardiovascular disease down the road.

There is some research to suggest that a high-fiber diet can help prevent colorectal cancer, although the evidence is not yet conclusive. High-fiber diets have also been connected to reducing your risk of breast cancer, as fiber helps to reduce levels of circulating estrogen, shares Tanya Zuckerbrot MS, RD, an NYC-based registered dietitian, who is also the founder of the F-Factor diet and a bestselling author.

Due to fiber's cleansing effects, it can help remove toxins in the blood, eliminating through your digestive process rather than your skin. Besides this, high-fiber foods tend to be high in antioxidants which can protect your skin from DNA-damaging free radicals.

Fiber's bulking properties can help you feel fuller, which promotes weight loss by creating a caloric deficit without hunger.

Printed in Great Britain
by Amazon